Mr Elasti

CW00968416

The Life and Poems of Sid Ozalid

Douglas John McLean Cairns

chipmunkapublishing
the mental health publisher

Douglas John McLean Cairns

Published by
Chipmunkapublishing
PO Box 6872
Brentwood
Essex CM13 1ZT
United Kingdom

http://www.chipmunkapublishing.com

Chipmunkapublishing gratefully acknowledge the support of Arts Council England.

Introduction

This book has been written to celebrate the work of The Artist Formally Known as Sid Ozalid, poet and tap dance teacher to the queen.

The work covers a period from 1977 to 2010. The only rule used to select the poems was that they had to have been performed live. You may also notice that several of the poems contain the word 'flea'.

The poems have been assembled in some sort of chronological order and to help put them into context I have sandwiched them between a short 'Sid' biography and a review from a show in London town.

This book is dedicated to my children, Kathy Bathy, Margot Fargo and Evie Weevie, all whom have the ability to fly.

I would also like to thank my darling wife, Anna Banana, without her love and support I would never have written this book or been able to walk in a straight line.

Love, Peace and Light

Douglas John McLean Cairns

Douglas John McLean Cairns

The proceeds from the sale of this book will be donated to the mental health charity Mind, for better mental health.

Mind campaigns vigorously to create a society that promotes and protects good mental health for all - a society where people with experience of mental distress are treated fairly, positively and with respect. www.mind.org.uk

Douglas John McLean Cairns

A Flock of Thistles

A flock of thistles with their bristles
Can fairly jab your thumb

But up your kilt the thistles' bristles
Will always jab your bum

**Unless you are wearing
Teflon non-stick underpants**

Douglas John McLean Cairns

Author Biography

Douglas fitted in very well at school until he had to learn something. Although having a vivid imagination his dyslexia went unnoticed in the Scottish school system of the late 1960s and early 1970s, resulting in him being bottom of most classes and leaving school with 'O' levels in Art and Technical Drawing. His teachers thought he was 'slow' and were happy as long as he did not chat in class. He chatted in class! They were not happy.

For most of his exams he would score less than 10% and was deeply ashamed of not being able to connect with what was going on around him, he watched lots of television or looked out of the window. He tried doing both at the same time, but this proved painful.

To help with his shyness and mumbling his parents sent him to elocution lessons and encouraged him to attend 'Children's Theatre'. Although primarily for bright, confident children, Douglas rarely missed a Saturday morning from the age of 9 to 16. He could never read from scripts but he was actively encouraged to improvise and express himself.

On leaving school at 16 he found employment working in the cartographic drawing office at BP in Aberdeen. He learned he could make a living by trying to do as he was told and working hard when he had to. His employers were happy as long as he did not chat all the time. He chatted all the time!

He found the structure of normal life puzzling and restrictive and was constantly challenged when having to fill in forms, write or talk in public. His solution was to invent his own character that would allow him to perform and express himself as he wished; in 1978 The Tap Dancing Poet Sid Ozalid was born.

As Sid, Douglas went on to perform for over 20 years on stage, radio and TV. Many people believe Sid to be some sort of madman, with his intense manic dancing and poetry. But to Douglas it was a perfect expression of himself and perhaps a way to release some of his childhood frustrations that were locked inside.

By the year 2000, for personal reasons, Douglas was no longer performing. He had thrown over 20 years of Sid memorabilia and material in the bin and cleared himself of many items from his past. He was separated from his wife and children and quickly became depressed.

Douglas' solution was to keep working harder. By this time he was head of Information Management for a major Oil and Gas company and had learned that by pushing both himself and others, he would be successful. He was wrong. The harder he pushed himself the worst it got.

He was asked to take time off work as his behaviour was upsetting to others. He was diagnosed with chronic depression. During this time he would often sleep for up to 20 hours a day. He was physically and mentally exhausted.

He found it difficult to talk; he needed help crossing the road and would often get lost or disorientated when walking to the shops. His mail would pile up and his phone would get cut off. He would hide in the corner of his room and cry. The pain inside was so bad he would cut his chest open to let it out. This did not work.

Douglas was very lucky that the company he worked for was supportive and gave him the required time to recover. The advice from his doctor was a mix of medication, rest, counselling and exercise. This was fully endorsed by his company doctor.

After an absence of six months Douglas went back to work part time and was amazed that some people would not talk to him and were vindictive and others found it easy and would offer support.

It would take a long time before Douglas could function fully in the work place. On his first day back he realised he did not know how to use the phone or switch his PC on. It was easier not to eat than own up to the fact that he could not function and was distressed and disorientated in the works restaurant.

He had to re-learn a number of fundamental skills, but with the help of a number of caring friends and colleagues he managed to get back to work and establish himself as a successful Facilitator, Change Manager and Behavioural Safety Expert.

He had to take care not to overwork himself, as he would often find himself dizzy and 'thinking in treacle' and had a short spell off work again in 2006. Since then he has got better and better at managing his 'illness'. Recognizing that prevention is preferable to cure, he lives by the maxim: look after yourself and do not be afraid of looking after others.

More recently Douglas has gone on a number of sponsored cycle rides and raised thousands of pounds for charity. He was very lucky to meet and marry a very nice lady and has slowly started writing and performing again, and as his friends say, they can tell when he is stable and his brain is opening up, and he starts being creative.

Contents

Douglas John McLean Cairns

First Bit
The Life of Sid Ozalid

Douglas John McLean Cairns

The Amazing Sid Ozalid

Legend has it that Sid Ozalid was born sometime during an eruption of earwigs. His father was thought to have been a redundant caveman and his mother a transvestite Egyptian monkey. Sid arrived on earth from the planet OZ in the year 1898. His spaceship was disguised as an old brown suitcase that was full of inflatable toys. His mission was to read from 'The Book Of Oz' and spread the word; the word may or may have not been 'mango'.

His talent as an entertainer first came to light in 1911, when he appeared with the Flying Ozalids. During this period he specialised in walking backwards into hat stands. Six years later he split from Flying Ozalids to form Sid and Sam the Ozalid Twins. This dynamic duo thrilled audiences with their routine entitled 'The First pickled Onion in Orbit', but alas this too came to an abrupt end due to lack of cupboard space.

Alternatively Sid's mother says that he was born in Glasgow, moved to the highlands of Scotland at the age of three, chased sheep for three years and arrived in Aberdeen in 1967. It is rumoured that she also says that he is a very silly but loveable boy, who was always a bit 'naive'.

He burst onto the Punk scene in 1978 as a one-legged tap dancing poet. Billed as 'The Tap Dancing Robert Burns' he would dance with his pet monkey, thrash himself with a daisy and beat his head with a tin tray. Some folks described him as a Punk Poet, but in reality he just happened to be a Punk who was performing poetry.

Dyslexia was the lens that helped Sid view the world,

the world of Laurel and Hardy, The Keystone Cops, Harpo Marx, Spike Milligan, and Wild Man Fisher. All first-class performers but touched by the ridiculous. As a young boy he lived in a vacuum of nonsense, watching the 'real' world go by, deciding that if you can't join them, enjoy yourself!

Punk gave him a window of opportunity to perform. He could be as ridiculous and silly as he wanted, some may say outrageous, but he was never ever rude.

Sid started off performing at local gigs round Aberdeen at salubrious establishments like The 62 Club, The Crescent Hotel, The Copper Beach, Ruffles Night Club, The Music Hall, Aberdeen University Union and Jay Jay's to name but seven.

Most of the time he would appear between the support and main act and strut his stuff. Performing his free-form wild dancing and whacking his tambourine in time with his poetry, he would intermittently pull out one of his inflatable toys. Ladies and Gentlemen 'Mickey the Monkey'. The audience always greeted the toys with great delight. Whether it was the introduction, or the quality of the toys we will never know.

Poems like 'Three Fat Ladies at the Bingo Hall', 'I'm In Love Said The Caterpillar' and 'Elephant in a Sack' had nothing to do with Punk, but their energy and disregard for norms fitted right in.

During this time he provided support for such acts as Simple Minds, The Clash, The Specials, OMD and many more, some of whom asked for him to be removed from the building.

He soon found himself travelling down to Edinburgh, Dundee and Glasgow, providing support at ever larger gigs. 'It was crazy, all I wanted to do was have fun and go and see a bunch of punk and new wave bands. Here I was getting my train fare paid, and getting into the gigs for free.'

In May 1979 he published Scotland's best selling postcard 'My Tortoise Can Burst Into Flames', a real favourite amongst young punks up and down Scotland. He also published a book of poems and songs, *The Book with Six Titles*, complete with self-styled drawings. This was further extended with his own fun page in Aberdeen's Fanzine *Granite City*.

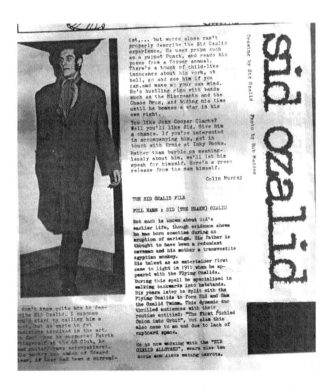

One Legged Tap Dancing Poet – Granite City

During 1979 and 1980 he was doing two or three gigs a week. If he was with the right audience he would go down a storm if he was with the wrong audience he would continue his act regardless of the strong encouragement to leave town, sometimes staying on longer just to endear himself further.

One of Sid's most pleasant memories was performing at Dundee Art Collage. 'It was a Dada movement, art and anti art. They had seen me performing at a very strange event in Edinburgh called The Electric Temple.' To begin with the audience of art students were very happy.

The first act consisted of a man in a white boiler suit walking on very slowly to some gentle music and psychedelic lighting; he carried a haversack on his back. On reaching the centre of the stage, he knelt down, took a typewriter out of the haversack and placed it in front of him. The audience were spell bound. Next came a mysterious parcel wrapped up in newspaper. The newspaper was unwrapped and a large fish appeared. The fish was fed into the typewriter and the man started to type on the fish'. Art or anti art?

A number of strange artistic acts followed. As the headliner, Sid sat in the audience with his friend Bob and Bob's wife Kate, who had sung in folk clubs during her youth and would 'like this sort of thing'.

As the evening went on a large number of leather-clad bikers turned up, whom, if not high on alcohol were crazy on the elixir of life. They hated the art students and, what some could call, pretentious performers. They took no time in letting everyone know of their displeasure. Things were getting very ugly as Sid left to get changed upstairs. He had to put on eight T-Shirts, three shirts, checked golfing trousers, a kilt, a curly wig and, last but not least, blow up his inflatable toys.

The promoter soon turned up and explained that fighting had broken out and Sid would not need to perform, but would still receive his full fee. Sid said he would like to go on and see how it went. As he walked down the dark and dusty staircase he was a bit surprised to see some of the bikers on stage fighting with the band that was trying to play.

'My lasting memory is seeing a crazy biker hit the bass player, take his guitar off him, and crack the poor man's head open as he wielded it like an axe.'

Once the bloodied band members had fled and the bikers were back in their seats, screaming for the next victim, up popped the Amazing Sid Ozalid. Sid danced faster than he had ever danced before, he hit himself on the head harder and faster than he had ever hit himself before, nailing his poetry like a machine gun, and the bikers loved him.

The cultural movement of Dadaism had begun in Zürich, Switzerland, in 1916 and was now alive and well in Dundee School of Art in 1979.

As an encore Sid was required to do his whole act all over again. He thought it wise to comply with the request. Bob's wife later suggested that next time Bob should attend the gig himself and she would stay home with their young son Greg. It had made her hair smell of cigarette smoke.

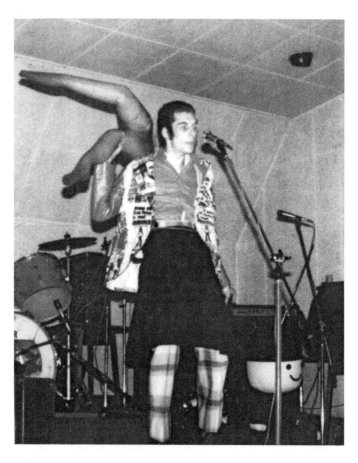

Douglas Hotel, Aberdeen 1978 supporting Another Pretty Face (The Waterboys)

The Electric Temple gigs were in Edinburgh, Glasgow and Amsterdam, although the Amsterdam gig never happened. Sid found this all a bit strange but the audience loved his mix of dancing and mad poetry, there were lots of dance groups, circus acts and a few bands thrown in for good measure.

'In Edinburgh the all-male dance group wore white thongs and covered themselves in talcum powder, I had never seen 20 men covering themselves in talcum powder before. It would appear that the best way to cover your body is to get another young man to do it for you. The dressing room was a fog of talc, and some older lady was complaining it would upset her snakes.'

The Snake Lady was also a big hit, she performed with her son. It looked as if they were beginning to perform after an absence of five years, as their costumes were far too small. She wore a black Basque and fish net stockings, and the son wore a cute assistant's outfit with gold trim that was half way up his arms and legs. The Snake Lady ate fire and covered herself in petrol. After some snake dancing and fire eating, she bent over, bursting out of her aged costume and placed an apple on the back of her neck. The son then produced a meat cleaver and nervously took aim at the apple. It was at this time that the audience became aware of the many scars and cuts on her neck. As they say 'practice makes perfect'.

At The Electric Temple gig in Glasgow, Sid met Clare Grogan, from a group called Altered Images. She had just appeared in the hit movie *Gregory's Girl* and been number 2 in the charts with 'Happy Birthday'.

'It was nice meeting someone famous; it was almost as good as my dressing room experience. Two girls from one of the dance groups came into my room. They had on skimpy outfits and started kissing and touching each other all over. After a few minutes they asked if I minded. "Not if you don't mind me blowing up my inflatable legs and life-size dolphin" I responded.'

'Apparently inflatable legs and dolphins are just the thing for attractive young dancing girls, the harder and faster I blew the faster and harder the girls kissed and embraced each other. I was not sure who would finish first, but I gave it all I had.'

As for the gig, Sid did get a very nice review in a national music magazine called *The Face*. 'Spike Milligan on magic mushrooms, spoo dee spoo doo'.

Sid liked the reference to Spike but had never experienced magic mushrooms and wondered why they had made the connection. His favourite quote had come from Aberdeen's *Peoples Journal*. 'Sid Ozalid: For anyone making a serious study into the totally ridiculous'.

Sid found that Ruffles nightclub in Aberdeen was a great place to pick up gigs. It was on the national tour route and lots of up and coming bands would perform. Jerry Dammers of The Specials thought Sid was tremendous and should come on tour with the band. The band told Jerry to stop being silly. A few months later The Specials and the Two Tone movement was dominating the British music scene.

'I supported a band called Wendy Woo and The Photos. The band enjoyed what I was doing and made their management take me down to London. Their album was Number 2 in the charts and I got all these ace gigs round London, and played to a thousand people at their end of tour gig in Brighton. Not bad for a daft boy with a suitcase full of toys.'

The reality was that Sid was being checked out by a number of agents and managers who could see he was a hit with the audience but had no idea what to do with him. The head of the Students Union Entertainment Conveners booked him to play at the Technical Collage in Glasgow. Due to the more than positive response, he booked him to play at the Conveners' yearly convention. This was full of booking agents, record companies and entertainment conveners from universities around the UK. Lots and lots of deals were done as the up and coming acts were showcased. Once again no one really knew what to do with Sid.

'I remember a long train journey down to Sheffield with my suitcase and staying in a B&B that served lovely bacon and egg. Attila the Stock Broker was at the gig. He was a nice man but was swearing all the time and kept talking about his record sales. Keith Allen (whose daughter Lilly went on to sell even more records than Attila the Stock Broker) was also on that night. He was also very good at swearing. In contrast I was dancing around with inflatable legs and singing a song about a Spanish Dustman with a Kipper round his Neck.'

Sid started performing with Jeremy Thom, as Sid and Sam the Ozalid Twins and later with his Legendary All-stars. In 1982 he released a musical book *Songs and Stories from a Suitcase Extravaganza*. This consisted of a six track EP and a forty page booklet of Sid's poems, songs and interesting drawings. Years later in 2007 Sid was asked to perform at an Ivor Cutler tribute concert. 'I was really embarrassed when folk kept coming up to me and telling me they had a copy of my record someplace at home. I thought the only ones who had a copy were Jeremy and my mum'.

In fact years earlier Sid had met Ivor in Edinburgh and over a cup of tea with scone and jam, had told Ivor that if he put the letter 'y' after each of his names it would spell Ivory Cutlery, very posh eating utensils that only came out when the Queen was visiting. Ivor asked Sid to leave the table. Sid was rather proud of his first and only 'spelling' joke.

Sam was good for Sid as he made him rehearse and provided structure and melody. Jeremy Thom is a very talented musician and, although having his own successful career in music, fitted right in with Sid's brand of fun.

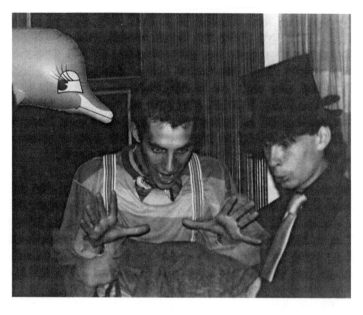

Sid and Sam the Ozalid twins with Daphne the Dolphin

Sid went on to perform at the Edinburgh Fringe, stunning audiences with shows such as 'My Granny's a Cowboy', 'I was a Teenage Xmas Tree' and 'Mr Elastic Brain'.

'The first few years were great fun, performing with Sam and the All-Stars was great, we would busk in the street and pull in a week's wage, much more than we would get at the door of the venue, but it helped pay the costs. The last year I did by myself. Alternative Comedy had arrived and it was lots more swearing and jokes about Margaret Thatcher. As I had never met Margaret Thatcher I stuck to my poems about mice, lice, toads and fleas.'

The Flying Ozalids were resurrected for the Fringe shows. 'I cannot remember much about it, apart from dressing up in tights. We had Darryl Thomson with us who would do some sort of escapology act as we performed. This consisted of Darryl being stripped naked and covered in jam, then live ants were placed into a sleeping bag and poor Darryl was tied up in the bag. '

'Each night the lads who were tying Darryl into the bag would make it tighter and tighter so he could not get out. Darryl would thrash around, song after song, poem after poem, silly dance after silly dance till he wriggled free. Some nice girl always felt sorry for him and took him home for chocolate cake and a healthy scrub down in the shower. I think that may be how he met his wife.'

During one of his visits to the festival Sid decided that he would run naked down Princes Street in nothing but a pair of pink socks and some trainers. The idea had come to him the previous week when he had taken part in a 10K 'Fringe' Fun Run around and over Arthur's Seat (a very large and beautiful hill in Edinburgh's Holyrood Park).

Sid entered the 10K race in a pair of pyjamas and a straight jacket, with balloons tied to his back. He had forgotten that you have to move your arms to run and found the very steep hill a bit harder than he first thought. Everyone thought he was a complete lunatic, but were very surprised to see him passing the majority of the runners on his way round the course.

On the outside he was a lunatic in a straight jacket who could hardly move, but on the inside he was a lunatic who could run a marathon in under three hours. Sid got himself a Top Ten finish and was the first costumed runner to finish, easily beating the four male nurses who were pushing a hospital bed.

Sid was proud of his 10K achievement. So proud of himself in fact that a week later he decided to run down Princes Street in support of wimps. Six foot two inches in height and under ten stone in weight he made the perfect wimp. Radio Forth thus decided to interview him.

The plan was that on the sound of the famous one o'clock cannon, Sid would set off from one end of Princes Street and run down to the other end and back again, all without being arrested.

Radio Forth wanted him on live, just before the one o'clock cannon and said they would order a taxi for Sid and drop him off in time for his run. Sid arrived at the radio station in his dressing gown and after answering some questions, set off in the taxi. All was going well till the taxi driver dropped him off and asked for the fare. Sid thought the Radio Station was going to pay, he had to show the driver that he was naked under the robe and had no money. Look I'm skint!

The run went well, the press turned up and true to his word Sid ran naked apart from a pair of pink socks and some trainers. The cannon fired at one o'clock, the robe fell and Sid set off with one of his socks pulled over his Willy. 'Me no daft me no silly me pull sock on to my Willy.'

Later in 1982 Sid was asked to support The Clash at Inverness Ice Rink. The Clash were due to have appeared in Aberdeen but their lead singer, Joe Strummer, had gone missing and the gig was cancelled and rescheduled in Inverness. Sid had met Joe in 1977 when The Clash were in Aberdeen during their White Riot Tour. Joe's trousers were falling down and Sid gave him a safety pin to keep them up.

Both Sid and local band apb were asked to perform support. Sid knew apb from performing with them at their first gig in Aberdeen at the Crescent Hotel. Since then they had become very successful and went on to record a Radio 1 session for John Peal. The crowd enjoyed apb and showed their appreciation by clapping and cheering, Sid and his All Stars got a mixed reaction. The people who did not like them spat at Sid, and the people who liked them spat at Sid. Punk was alive and well in Inverness. Sid was sent to the dry cleaners.

Abp went on to further success, primarily in the US having their records played on college radio and in hip New York clubs such as Danceteria, Berlin and the Mudd Club. They went on to support James Brown and are still highly regarded. Sid never got his safety pin back from Joe Strummer and never had his record played in hip New York clubs.

Around the same time the Saturday morning children's TV program *Tiswas* was about to lose its main stars: Chris Tarrant, Lenny Henry and John Gorman. They had started work on *O.T.T* a late night version of *Tiswas* intended for an adult audience. In support of this new enterprise they tried to see Sid at the Edinburgh Fringe but could not find the venue. They then tried to see Sid in Dundee, when they were in town along with Sally James performing as The Four Bucketeers. The times of their shows clashed so Sid was left to move things forward with John Gorman.

Gorman had been a member of The Scaffold, best known for their 1968 hit single Lilly the Pink. As a child Sid had spent hours dancing to Lilly the Pink in his bedroom. Now over ten years later Sid asked if he could come and play the violin on a lobster and be wrapped in cling film and smoke a cigarette through a rubber hose. Gorman was open to all the ideas and invited Sid down to perform in London. At first Sid was excited at the prospect until it became clear that he would be expected to travel down to London every week if he were to be a regular on the show.

Sid declined, 'I loved the idea of playing the violin on a lobster. I would get tingly inside each time I came up with an idea that they liked, but I had no need to travel down there every week. London was too big, too noisy and I felt overwhelmed at the idea. One show would be great, but week after week'.

As Sid's mum had said many times before, he was a very silly but loveable boy, who was always a bit 'naive'.

'I watched all the O.T.T shows and liked the guy they had booked, called Alexei Sayle, it just never felt right for me to take it any further.'

Chris Tarant went on to be a household name in the UK and ultimately hosted *Who wants to be a Millionaire*, Sid never playing the violin on a lobster.

The window of Punk opportunity was closing, music and youth culture had moved on, Sid would have to look for other opportunities to enjoy performing.

In January 1984 he auditioned and was invited to perform on two different talent shows. Once again the producers liked what Sid was doing but did not know how to describe him. They settled for 'eccentric'.

First up was BBC Scotland's *Stars in your Eyes* hosted by Janet Brown, who had been married to the *Carry On* actor Peter Butterworth who had also appeared in *Dr Who*. In Sid's eyes this made Janet a comedy goddess.

Sid drove his suitcase down to Glasgow and did some impersonations of famous peoples' clothes, including Marlon Brando's jacket and Joan Collins' dress. This was coupled with the fine poem 'Has anyone seen Mrs Polytheyn'. Despite his energy and elastic movements the judges were not impressed, but Janet loved him and kept popping in and out of his dressing room. Sid took home some paper cups with the BBC Logo on them. They were not to be used when independent TV channels were being watched.

Sid expected he would come in last, and as it was down to a postal vote from viewers, he decided to vote for himself. He sent off 150 postcards, using the money from well-paying student union gigs to pay for the stamps. The following week, he was a bit surprised to find out that he had won and had to go back for the all-winners show.

For the *Stars in your Eyes* final he unleashed his impersonations of famous buildings: The Eiffel Tower, The Post Office Tower, The Tay Bridge and Tay Bridge Disaster. He also performed a fine rendition of a poem called 'Family Tricks'. This time it was just down to the judges. He came in a splendid last!

Next up was *The Fame Game* with Granada TV, hosted by Tim Brooke-Taylor, who had appeared in *The Goodies* and whose grandfather had played centre forward for England. Sid liked the Goodies and this time set off on an aeroplane to Manchester. Not being a seasoned traveller, Sid was very sick on the flight and had to be helped from the plane on arrival.

The ground crew would not let him leave the airport until they thought he was capable of looking after himself. He was held in the airport for over two hours, the plus point being that Sid saw the world famous Scotland and Manchester United football player Denis Law walk past him in the airport. 'Wait till Tim Brooke-Taylor hears about this,' Sid thought to himself as he whispered to a plastic flower arrangement in the airport lounge.

Things only got better at Granada as Sid met Jim Bowen from the world famous *Bullseye* TV program and was shown round the set of *Coronation Street*.

Sid did not get to meet Tim Brooke-Taylor as all the acts were recorded on separate days. Sid loved it as he had a nice large audience to perform to, he went down well and was on for over 20 minutes, he was only to do 2 minutes, but both he and the audience were having a good time. The producers used Sid's impersonations of seagulls: Seagull at a wedding, seagull at a library, seagull dying in flight. He lost!.

In the late 1990s Sid got another chance to meet Denis Law and played football with him in the car park of Grampian TV. Denis had no idea who Sid was but was very polite and later showed Sid how to drink red wine.

Sid made it back to Manchester a few months after recording the *Fame Game*, when he was performing at both the Manchester and Salford universities. He was to stay in the halls of residence, but Sid was delighted when one of the nice staff from Granada turned up for one of his shows. She was a very pleasant lady who invited Sid to stay at hers for a sleep over.

Sid was carrying his suitcase every ware he went and was pleased to see that she had a car. She also had a three-bedroom house. Sid was offered a cup of tea and some chocolate biscuits. He was more than happy to accept. He was then offered a choice of drugs from a rather posh teak box. Sid declined, as he had never taken drugs before. His hostess enjoyed her drugs and Sid enjoyed his chocolate biscuits. Sid was in for a further surprise when it was time for bed. He had a choice of rooms, one of the choices involved sharing with the nice young lady.

Sid chose the spare room and another packet of chocolate biscuits. He woke up happy in the morning but covered in crumbs. The nice lady had to leave for work.

Around 1986 Sid went on to perform with a man called George Norvell. George had lots of nice hi-tech guitars and gadgets and the two of them tried out a number of routines that George then recorded into backing tracks. The audience were a bit confused; they could hear a full band, with heavy drum and bass lines, so expected a real band with a real drummer, if not then they were being cheated. How times change.

Sid used the sound tracks to record a video *A Bag Full of Donkeys*. They were also invited to perform at the Locomotion in Paris, part of the world famous Moulin Rouge. They were invited to perform as part of a Scottish theme night that was headlined by Gaelic rock band Runrig. Sid was a good friend of their manager, Marline Ross; this would explain why he got the gig.

The youthful French audience were enjoying the unusual dancing and rhyming experience in time with hi-tech music, until George's gadget combination blew the PA system. This did not put Sid off, he danced his little Gaelic heart out and performed the rest of the act in pigeon French. The organisers should not have been surprised at the PA incident as they had first seen Sid perform in Glasgow University, where his pyrotechnics had set off the fire alarms and the building had to be evacuated. Eight hundred students went out and over a thousand happy Glaswegians came back in.

Sid used the backing tracks and started working with Gerry 'Bongo' Dawson. Gerry was a jolly trumpet player who would be out most nights of the week blowing his own trumpet for money. The two spent a bit of time in London town, performing in comedy clubs. Sid was once hit in the face with a full bottle of beer, that someone had thrown from the audience. A stunned Sid could not believe it. Who would be mad enough to throw a full bottle? In Scotland they have the sense to drink it first. Sid thanked the audience very much and drank the beer. This was after inviting the 'guilty' individuals outside to discuss the issue further. They politely declined.

Robbie the Pict, invited them to perform at a Pictish Festival in Letham, the village is famous for 'The Girdlestane', a Pictish monument, looking towards Dunnichen Hill. There are also some shops, including a grocery which incorporates the post office and newsagent, a school, a bakery and a hairdresser.

Over a 1000 folk descended on the lovely village, many of them dressed as Picts from the 10th century, who had stopped the Roman's from invading Scotland. Sid received a mixed audience response. The folks down the front who were wearing dead pheasants on their heads could relate with Sid's antics and wanted more and more. The musical purists who had been pushed to the back were not impressed with electronic backing tracks and crazy leg dancing. Everyone loved Gerry Bongo and his magic trumpet.

Sid and Gerry also made it to the Shetland Rock festival. Sid met up once again with Toxik Ephex, regarded by many as one of Scotland's best-ever punk bands. Sid had first met their guitarist Fred 'Inspector Blake' Wilkinson in the early 1980s.

'Sam and I were doing a gig at Jay Jay's at the beach with the All Stars and the Flying Ozalids. During the break, young Fred came up and asked me to plug his weekend gig. I was happy to do so but could not remember the name of his band and had to ask about ten times during my act, so think he got a lot of publicity.'

Supporting Sid that night, were some other young men who had met him at a jumble sale and asked him for a gig. He was impressed as they had a drum machine and a drum synth (a drum pad). They were called 'Alone Again Or'. Sid would see one of the young men on a regular basis, as Sid went for his daily run round the grounds of Westburn Park close to Cornhill Hospital in Aberdeen. Sid was training for one of his many marathons and young Colin Angus was on his lunch break. Alone Again Or went on to become The Shamen, who had a worldwide hit with 'Ebeneezer Goode' and a double platinum selling album *Boss Drum*. Sid went on to give his running shoes away to a blind grandmother with big feet and got himself a secondhand bike. Colin always said hello to Sid in the street and Sid always asked him about the secret of the magic drum pad you hit with a stick.

The journey up to Shetland for the Rock Festival was by overnight North Sea Ferries. Sid was still not a good traveler and spent all night Sellotaped to his bunk as Gerry Bongo passed his trumpet round the different members of Toxik Ephex.

Prior to going on the boat journey Sid had been interviewed by Northsound Radio, who were keen to hear all about the bands that were playing. Sid offered up his Famous Building impersonations. Being on the radio this forced the young radio presenter, Mark Findlay, to describe the impersonations to his listeners. Sid and Mark hit it off and Sid was invited as a regular guest on Mark's show. This soon developed into a full hour once a week called 'Invisible Radio'. Mark was a happening young DJ around town and Sid would come in and give live cooking lessons to Mark or give reviews on swimming pools and ice-cream parlors he had visited over the weekend.

Sid's popularity on Mark's show grew amongst the young audience of Aberdeen. At this time his mother thought he was thirty three, Sid thought he was a hundred and three and most of their radio audience thought he was around thirteen.

Sid and Mark started getting more fan mail than the rest of the full time DJs put together. This was mainly down to Sid re-inventing the postcard trick. Most of the show revolved round the bizarre mail the two of them received. Mark was over the moon at such popularity from his audience and Sid was over the moon that his letter writing skills were such a big hit with Mark. To be fair, Sid mostly encouraged his friends and family to write in on his behalf. At Christmas time they had a show that spanned over two nights, called 'The Unfortunate Turkey Show'. They played summer hits and sat in their swimming trunks with the lights turned up full. Sid got to sing all his own jingles and his best and only mate Abby Donian, played by Alex Lovie would phone in with the latest sports news. Sid's mum would sing as his mother-in-law played the piano and Giorgio the Poet would lay down some rhythm and rhyme.

One of Sid's biggest fans at the station was Richard Gordon, who gave the real sports reports. Richard was a regular contributor to Sid's mail sack but always under a different name. Richard thought he was competing with real mail from listeners and tried each week to achieve 'letter of the week'. Richard went on to become anchor man for Radio Scotland's football coverage and his voice is known to hundreds of thousands of Scots on sports days.

Mark also left and went on to become Head Of Music at Capital Radio. He was replaced on Invisible Radio by Dave McLeod who co-presented with Sid till 1992. Like Jeremy Thom before him Dave provided structure. Dave was a talented actor, musician and DJ in his own right, but worked well with Sid and provided him with an opportunity to be creative and perform.

Dave subsequently left to become the voice of Channel 4 as a continuity announcer. Millions across the UK now hear his voice and he has an extensive collection of woolen cardigans.

At no time did Sid ever think that the people he was working with were going on to be successful in the entertainment business and leaving him behind. Perhaps he should have, but he was just happy to have a window of opportunity to create and share his own brand of fun.

Sid wrote and co-presented *Invisible Radio* from 1988 – 1992, one show a week for over four and a half years. During this time The Lemon Tree opened its doors in Aberdeen and commissioned Sid to write and produce *Invisible Radio* on stage. This was a chance to bring all the characters from the radio show to life. Sid said yes to the kind offer. Then along with Dave McLeod and Alex Lovie had to work out how to create them for a live audience. They got lots and lots of help.

Seeing is Believing was the first show, followed by *Life on a Stick*. 'I was very lucky that I had so many good people to work with. Our support team from Northsound Radio was first class, although I do not think the boss knew how much time his staff were spending on helping us.'

Sid was right that the directors of the station found it hard to understand why he was on the radio, but they could not argue with the fan mail. If only they had known that 90% of it came from Sid himself.

The Lemon Tree went very well. Sid's children could come to see him on stage for the first time and the cast were pleasantly surprised that the audience consisted of complete families, grandparents, parents and children. Sid's poetry and dance spanned over three generations.

Dave moved to London after their last live, stage show *Mad, Bad and Bald*. Sid took to growing giant sunflowers in his back garden. A few months later the two of them would be paired up again when Sid was asked to present a show for Grampian TV. Tern Television were commissioned to make a program about the Aberdeen Alternative Festival and approached Sid to present the show. Sid was happy as long as he got to write it and invite his friend along to take part. Tern TV agreed and the result was a thirty minute show called *The Idiots Guide to the Aberdeen Alternative Festival.* The program was short listed for an award. It lost!.

Sid was no stranger to TV; after his experience on the talent shows, he had picked up a lot of work as an extra, appearing with and meeting a number of household names. In 1989 Den Watts played by Leslie Grantham had just been 'killed off' from the ITV soap opera *Eastenders.* Leslie was front page news at the time and one of TV's biggest stars. His next TV program was called *Winners and Losers* and was filmed in Glasgow. Sid got to play a very small part as a TV presenter at a boxing match. He was very pleased to sit next to ex-world champion boxer Jim Watt. 'The best bit was at lunchtime when I went to get a coffee and 'Dirty Den Watts' asked if I wanted milk and poured it for me. Wow what a day. He also had a chat with my wife on the phone, I never saw her again.'

Sid went on to portray mass murderer 'Denis Neilson' on a Channel 4 program called *Evil.* He even spent two days 'making out' with an attractive young lady in a program that stared James Fox.

'The character James was playing was having an affair and during a scene in a restaurant dance club, they wanted to create tension between the 'cheating' characters who were out with their spouses by having young lovers in the background. I got to be one of the young lovers, but filming carried over to a second day. The next day we both turned up with extra strong mints as the continuity girl got us back into position. I did try my attractive young female partner with some poems but she just told me to get on with it.'

Sid had also appeared in an advert for Tenants Lager. They had a new advertising campaign with the slogan

'Iv Got Mine'. It was shown as the first advert of the New Year in 1990. The advert involved a fisherman arriving home from sea on his fishing boat, walking into the pub to meet his mates and having a drink of Tenants Lager. Sid was amongst a group of extravagant extras who had been employed to dress up as fishermen and stand around drinking beer with foam on top to make it look good. A young piano player had been chosen to play the part of the fisherman's crewmate who would throw him his bag from the boat up to the peer; the fisherman would catch the bag, give a wave and head straight into the warm pub.

Unfortunately the swell of the sea was rather heavy and the boat kept going up and down. The poor piano player was getting tiered and could not throw the bag up to the waiting fisherman. Sid was chosen instead and was happy to throw a 'hold all' full of newspapers up to the waiting fisherman. After the shot Sid changed his yellow waterproofs for a nice woolen jumper his mother-in-law had knitted him for Xmas. He looked so warm and friendly he was chosen to be one of the fisherman's mates who welcomed the returning hero into the pub. One second Sid was on the boat throwing the bag and the next he was in the pub drinking larger with extra foam on top. Sid felt rather proud of himself, but although managing to appear in two places at the same time, he only got paid the once.

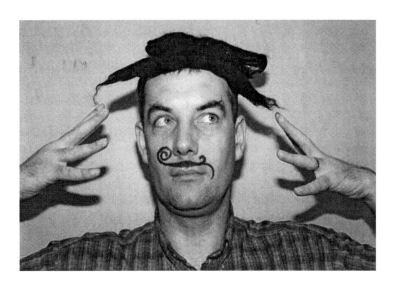

By the early 1990s and Sid was spending more and more time in his garden and was thinking of getting himself a pet monkey. *Invisible Radio* was no longer on air, and the opportunities to perform were getting less and less. Sid had been getting told for years that if he wanted to develop and move on in his career he would have to move to London and establish himself in the Comedy Circuit. He had a wife and two young children and was not about to leave them to starve to death as he danced around London with an inflatable dolphin strapped to his chin. The London opportunity had come and gone ten years earlier with the opportunity with O.T.T. Since then he had been to London and performed at the world famous 'Comedy Store' plus an assortment of gigs at various comedy clubs. He did not enjoy the noise, the traffic or the tube. He was happy to enjoy the 'odd' performance without having to running away to join the circus or filling his underpants full of goldfish.

Sid spent more and more time with his children and talking to his plants, but there was no rest for the lunatic fringe. In 1996 a man called Paddy Burns opened a comedy club in Aberdeen, called 'Open Mics'. He approached Sid to MC the club. Sid declined as he was planning to expand from giant sunflowers to wild summer flowers and electric bubble wrap. Paddy explained that it would just be for two weeks till he got a real MC. Sid agreed, performing under his real name 'Doogalie Woogalie is a go–go' and soon ended up running the club. Sid renamed it 'The Laughing Carrot', opened a second club in Dundee and the two weeks turned into two years.

'It was fun. I got to meet a bunch of good folks who were moving up the comedy ladder. I was invited to perform at the Dundee Rep and Perth Theatre. I could take my puppets along and do whatever I felt liked, and provided a platform for local talent trying their luck.' Sid did book a number of up and coming acts. He booked ex-Butlin's Redcoat, Johnny Vegas' for £50. 'One week he had drunk two bottles of red wine and was throwing up in our sink and the next week he was all over the TV and press'.

By the end of 1998 Sid decided to stop performing. His third child was due to arrive and he wanted to be around more to enjoy her growing up. He was back on the radio and travelling most weeks for gigs. 'All my children have the ability to fly, I just wanted to be around to see the first few flights'. Little did he know that divorce and depression was round the corner carrying a black bag with his name on it.

People had always told Sid he was mad. He thought they were joking until the dawning of the new millennium, suddenly he had a doctor's certificate to prove what people had been telling him for years.

Not only did Sid stop performing he stopped writing, after years of doing his own thing and expressing himself in all sorts of crazy ways his body and brain would not function.

The best cure for madness is a stable routine, lots of fresh air, exercise and counselling. Sid got himself a new bike and cycled across the Sinai Desert. He then cycled round Cuba, along the Great Wall of China, down the West Coast of India and though Jordan to the Red Sea. The fresh air and exercise helped. He got out of the house more and invested in a digital camera.

After a number of years Sid performed a number of fund raising concerts for Mind, the Mental Health Charity, under the name ' The Artist Formally Known As Sid Ozalid'.

In 2005 he performed at the Aberdeen Arts Centre along with 85-year-old Poetry Slam Champion Hilda Meers, and poet songwriter Steve Webb as the 'Talking Handbags'. Once again Sid performed under his own name of 'Doogalie Woogalie is a go–go'. The fourth handbag was the highly regarded Sculptress, Janet McEwen, who broadly explored gender issues by decided to play with the handbag as a symbol / metaphor for the often contradictory cultural views of woman: as both vessel and burden.

Sid had no real interest in ever performing again. His focus was on regaining his health. He had met and married a very nice lady and was looking forward to cycling to the moon.

With the encouragement of his youngest daughter and with the support of his wife, Sid started performing again in 2010. He has taken it one step at a time and made sure that he both stretches and enjoys himself. His shows in London, Amsterdam and Aberdeen have all being well received. He has also been in the recording studio with Iain Slater from apb. Iain had gone on to work as the sound engineer for Dutch rock band Kane and more recently Pete Docherty. Iain makes Sid behave himself when they work together. Sid says 'people may or may not like the material we are recording, but one thing is sure. The quality of the recording is first class.'

Sid has six bikes, is now only slightly interesting and lives in a shoe.

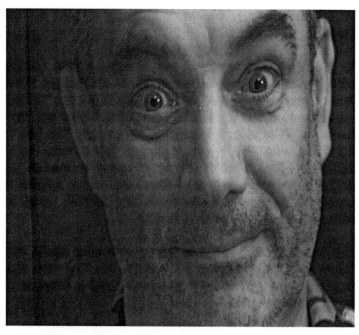

The Artist sometimes known as Sid Ozalid

Second Bit

The Poems of Sid Ozalid

1977 to 2010

Douglas John McLean Cairns

Three Ladies at the Bingo Hall

Three fat ladies at the bingo hall
They didn't win started a brawl
Policeman came arrested them all
Three fat ladies at the bingo hall

Down at the station behind the bars
They were taken there in three police cars
Three fat ladies in the nick
Handbags full of a half brick

My visions going hazy
My mind is going crazy
Just thrash me with a daisy
Oh Yea Oh Yea
Just thrash me with a daisy
Oh Yea

Three fat ladies at the back of the bus
Couldn't pay their fare started a fuss
Conductors name it was Russ
Three fat ladies at the back of the bus

Darby and Jones Club they were all there
To say a word they wouldn't dare
Three fat ladies would fill them in
Three fat ladies all drink gin

My visions going hazy
My mind is going crazy
Just thrash me with a daisy
Oh Yea Oh Yea
Just thrash me with a daisy
Oh Yea

Three fat ladies in their Sunday best
Feathered hats woolly vest
Three fat ladies in the nick
Handbags full of a half brick

My visions going hazy
My mind is going crazy
Just thrash me with a daisy
Oh Yea Oh Yea
Just thrash me with a daisy
Oh Yea

My Mothers name is Mazy
Her cat is very lazy
Just thrash me with a daisy
Oh Yea Oh Yea
Just thrash me with a daisy
Oh Yea

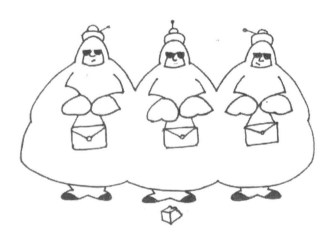

The Tale of Two Tailor's Dummies

The tailor's dummy's legs
Were swinging too and fro
To stop this terrible swinging
He tied them in a bow

The tailor he was angry
For his dummy had no sense
Last week he'd gone quite mad
Was nervy tired and tense

The dummy's name was Willy
He had an easy life
But that day he had been battered
By his dear and loving wife

She was a dummy of great stature
A curve in ever stitch
Despite her smooth flannels
She had a nervous twitch

She used to twitch so badly
It made her rant and rave
Willy used to tell her
It would send her to the grave

She twitched and said to Willy
Now listen here my lad
Don't you answer back to me again
You know it makes me mad

With those very words
She hit him on the chin
With one almighty shove
She shoved him in a bin

Now Willy stays inside that bin
His legs swing too and fro
Whenever he gets lonely
He ties them in a bow.

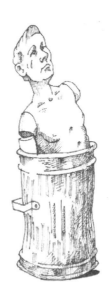

Family Tricks

My best friend raises octopus
I like licking slates
Auntie nibbles armchairs
Mother swallows plates

Sister plays accordion
Father's crushing peas
Brothers munching light bulbs
Granny's smoking fleas

These pastimes may sound silly
We call them family tricks
Something that comes naturally
Like eating Weetabix

Douglas John McLean Cairns

L Sid

L Sid you were a hero
L Sid you were so great
L Sid you wrestled poodles
Like a fish lies on a plate

L Sid you were so gruesome
Mighty big and strong
Spoke with the same aggression
As a nightingale sings its song

L Sid your sword was very sharp
Your armour shiny bright
Riding into battle
Like a penguin flies at night

When the fighting was over
The battles they were won
You went home and rested
Until the invention of the gun

I'm In Love Said the Caterpillar

I'm in love said the caterpillar
He said it to the flea
I'm in love said the caterpillar
Why can't you be in love with me?

Why … Can't … You … Be … In … Love … With …
Me?

I've wrapped myself inside my cocoon
I'm staying in there
I'll come out soon
Come round to your house
Fly around
Brand new wings
Won't make a sound
When I come back
It'll be for a day or two
I know that it's worth it
I would do anything for you

I'm in love said the caterpillar
He said it to the flea
I'm in love said the caterpillar
Why can't you be in love with me?

Why … Can't … You … Be … In … Love … With …
Me?

Don't talk to the ant
With the red crew cut
He ain't cool

I'm the boy around here
I'm moving it
I'm doing it

Douglas John McLean Cairns

Like a crawling
Flying
Love machine

I'm in love said the caterpillar
He said it to the flea
I'm in love said the caterpillar
Why can't you be in love with me?

Why ... Can't ... You ... Be ... In ... Love ... With ...
Me?

Coloured Braces

When I was young I had no fun
Always lost the races
Now I'm old I am bold
I wear coloured braces

Tie them round the starting post
Ping myself away
Everybody stands right back
Fastest race all day

One day I'll join the army
Sign my life away
March around look real smart
Kill gorillas every day

Polish up me buttons
Gun and bayonet too
Don't think I'd kill gorillas
Just feed them poisoned peanuts at the zoo

Douglas John McLean Cairns

When my bedtime demons grab me

I'll ping them in the face

A pair of coloured braces

Saviour of the human race

Stepping Out

I stepped out of the oven
First time in weeks
Warm but cramped rent is cheap
Electricity never leaks

Asked a girl back to my place
Game of cards and some bridge
She couldn't have been promiscuous
Spent all night in the fridge

My tortoise Can Burst Into flames

I look into your eyes and it reminds me, of the first time

I saw my tortoise burst into flames

My tortoise can burst into flames
He's really cool and picks up dames
Knows what he likes
He likes party games
My tortoise can burst into flames

Your nipples are like a stampede of ants

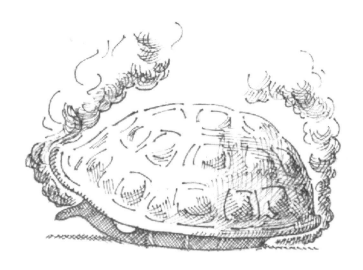

Down At The Farm (What's Going On)

What's going on down at the farm
It's all good fun, won't do you any harm
Better watch that dog, it may bite your arm
What's going on down at the farm

The cow is doing summersaults
The farmers going blind
The beggar loves a donkey
He is good and he is kind

The dog is in the tractor
The haystack's in the well
The beggar loves a donkey
He likes to make a smell

Ten mice are running backwards
There is bacon in the tent
The beggar loves a donkey
But never pays his rent

The pig it is metallic
The sheep they are dyed blue
The beggar loves a donkey
If you saw it so would you

The hen looks like a turnip

The barn has blown away

The beggar loves a donkey

It is a sunny day!

Blaa ... blaa ... blaa ... blaa

Blaa ... blaa ... blaa ... blaa

Blaa ... blaa ... blaa ... blaa ... Blaa!

Lovebirds

I know a Spanish dustman with a kipper round his neck
Singing songs to Freddie who's on the lower deck
Sailing off on holiday a month off in the sun
Freddie's getting lonely writes home to his mum
For they are …
ooh ooh ooh ooh ooh Lovebirds

Land on a lonely island, blue skies all around
Unloading their baggage they hear a funny sound
Scouring round the island they find footsteps in the sand
Dustman's feeling dizzy Freddie holds his hand
For they are …
ooh ooh ooh ooh ooh Lovebirds

Then a girl called Joseph carves initials on a tree
That makes the dustman happy Freddie shouts 'that makes us three'
Pam tree plays a saxophone Freddie starts to dance
Dustman's feeling happy with a goldfish down his pants
For they are …
ooh ooh ooh ooh ooh Lovebirds

The sounds of tram wheels turning cause a startle in their eyes

It is only an illusion really no surprise

Until a hairy guinea pig gave them money to go away

Now that hairy guinea pig regrets that very day

For they are …

ooh ooh ooh ooh ooh Lovebirds

Lovebirds are groovy

Lovebirds can dance

Lovebirds are happy

With goldfish in their pants

Mortgage and Cortina Syndrome

Mortgage and Cortina syndrome
Mortgage and Cortina life
Mortgage and Cortina syndrome
Two point two and one wife

Watching Albert on the TV
Sitting in his armchair
His degree is in his pocket
All grey hairs are well hid

The lawn mower is well adjusted
Plugging in the mouse trap
Hanging out his bedroom window
He is just a crimplene kid

You'll never get his cashmere jersey
Polishing the mantelpiece
Three Alsatians and one hamster
Never tell you what he did

The saxophone is bright and briskly
Flying to a foreign land
The plastic gnome is for sale
Clip on waterproof teapot lid

Mortgage and Cortina syndrome
Mortgage and Cortina life
Mortgage and Cortina syndrome
Two point two and one wife

Red-eared Seagull

It's a red-eared seagull's life for me

Said half a kangaroo

To the other half called Lee

I don't really know said Lee

I quite fancy being

A blue-legged Egyptian flea

Tupperware Health Food Day

Shredded shoe
Like shredded wheat
Is very good to eat

Old brown boot
With lentil soup
Is messy on the feet

Plastic bag
With Worchester sauce
Is high on vitamin A

Porridge oats
With a screw on top
It's a Tupperware Health Food Day

Singing ...
Dummy dum
Dum dummy dum day
Dummy dum
Dum dummy dum day
Dum dum dummy
Dummy dum day
Dum dum dummy day

Douglas John McLean Cairns

Dum dum dummy
Dummy dum day

It's a Tupperware Health Food Day

Come Into My party

Come into my party
Step into my house
The banjo is playing
Being strummed by a mouse

Mother is screaming
Beethoven is dead
I hear his music
Going round in my head

The mongrel's in the greenhouse
Laughing at the plants
The joke's on his legs
He gets eaten by red ants

I know he's got a telescope
Giggles in the rain
Ants are still eating
He giggles on in pain

The party's nearly over
The mongrel rushes out

Beethoven plays louder

Mother starts to shout

The party's in tatters

There's a moral here to tell

Mother stood on the red ants

The dog's name was Nell

Twenty-five Tons of Ferret Dropping

Walk and talk like Sexton Blake
Throw yourself into a lake
Just an ugly caricature
Never too late never too sure
Say that it is groovy
Say that it is fine
Say that when your shaving
It's raining all the time
You know I go superstore shopping
There's nothing quite the same as …
Twenty-five tons of ferret dropping

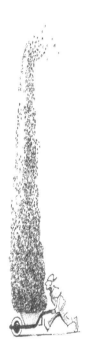

Working class hero
With nothing to say
Don't know where you're going
But go anyway
Rather sing about pygmies
Than sing about life
Love Yogie bear
He loves his wife
Like a waste-paper bin
A product of sin
Old banana peel
Baked bean tin
Three-legged race
The hare is still hopping
There's nothing quite the same as …
Twenty-five tons of ferret dropping

Douglas John McLean Cairns

Just a young man
Without any age
Keeps common sense
Locked up in a cage
Navy blue bloomers
Hanging on the line
Clash with your eyes
Can't be mine
Lorry the lobster
Sitting on his bike
Knows a monkey
His name is Mike
Lilac pig
Takes one hell of a stopping
There's nothing quite the same as …
Twenty-five tons of ferret dropping

The Vicar's Pet Shop

See the vicar against the tree
He lifts his leg and he kicks me
Kicks me

If you keep monkeys in a cage
It makes the vicar in a rage
He won't die of old age
If you keep monkeys in a cage

Do you like dogs or cats or rats
Lie down on grass or lie on mats
Do you wear boots do you wear hats
Do you like dogs or cats or rats

I see a goldfish on the floor
I pick it up and eat it
Some people think it is a joke
Me I just don't get it

The cat sat on the mat
So what do you think of that
The cat sat everywhere it went
That's why the cat was fat

The rabbit hops the rabbit skips
The rabbit with the squiggly hips
Don't draw on him with felt pens
Don't keep batteries inside hens

See the vicar against the tree
He lifts his leg and he kicks me
Kicks me

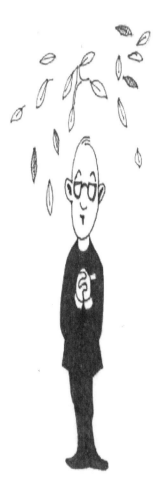

Mosquito's wing

Give me your mosquito's wing
Promise you I won't sing
Might even do a highland fling
If you give me your mosquito's wing

Mosquito's wing just give it me
Not the wing of a Bumble Bee
Mosquito's wing is very wee
Mosquito's wing give it me

Bzzz bzzz bzzz bzzz bzzz
Mosquito's wing
Is very wee
Bzzz bzzz bzzz bzzz bzzz
Mosquito's wing
Give it me

Catch a falling sputnik
Put it in a meat pie
Drive the red bus away
Drive it round the corner
Straight into a lamppost
Does the lady love Milk Tray?

Douglas John McLean Cairns

Give me your mosquito's wing
Promise you I won't sing
Might even do a highland fling
If you give me your mosquito's wing

Mosquito's wing just give it me
Not the wing of a Bumble Bee
Mosquito's wing is very wee
Mosquito's wing give it me

I Am Just A Budgie

I am just a budgie
Sitting on a perch
You don't even like me
You hit me with a stick

One day when it was beautiful
My mother laid an egg
Out of it came my brother
Who bit me on the leg

The old man wore green trousers
And when they were up they were up
And when they were down they were down
And when they were only half way up

He got arrested
Most unfortunate

Gertrude Zip-Ding

Gertrude Zip-Ding is a very strange name
It belongs to a girl who stands in the rain
She imitates puddles and floats down the drain
Gertrude Zip-Ding is a very strange name

She has a dog she likes it you can tell
It's been dead three weeks and beginning to smell
It bit the postman and will go to hell
Gertrude Zip-Ding doesn't feel too well

Gertrude doesn't feel too well
Gertrude doesn't feel too well
Gertrude Zip-Ding doesn't feel too well

She has a bike she likes it you can tell
Cycled through the river and fell down the well
Began to drown as she rang her bell
Gertrude Zip-Ding doesn't feel so swell

She has a head she likes it you can tell
Fell off the other day at the bottom of the well
It bit the dog who began to smell
Gertrude Zip-Ding doesn't feel too well

Gertrude doesn't feel too well

Gertrude doesn't feel too well

Gertrude Zip-Ding doesn't feel too well

Elephant In A sack

Undertaker
Lorry maker
Next-door neighbour
Mr Baker

Wear your raincoat
When it rains
Close your blinds
And windowpanes

The rain goes
Split splot splat
My mother's getting fat

The rain goes
Split splot sploo
Hear a cow go moo

Hundreds of little elephants
Run around in hats
Rain it is still falling
The size of cricket bats

Bathtubs are filling
Terrapins run away
Wise owl says
The sun's been painted grey

Mr Elastic Brain

Galoshes spring a leak
Tie your elephant in a sack
With a piece of rubber hosing
Give it a good whack

When the storm is over
The rains have gone away
No one seems to know
Where the elephant lay

Elephant Elephant in a sack
Turn around and don't come back ... don't come back

Douglas John McLean Cairns

My Friend the Toad

Walking and talking
Dining with lice
Nobody likes him
In fact he's not nice

He's got a green face
His eyes stick out
His skin is wet
They think he's a lout

Lying in mud
And slime all day
If they could catch him
They'd take him away

Spots on his back
Lumps on his cheeks
He always croaks
He never squeaks

He's my friend
The Toad the Toad the Toad

He's my friend

The Toad the Toad the Toad

Got squashed on the road

My friend the Toad

Shopping List (and a half pound of cheese please)

Here is my shopping list
Bag full of money
Come to get the shopping
Give it to my mummy

Half a pound of bacon
Bag full of nails
Slimy custard
Assorted rats tails
Crispy carrots some dead fleas
And a half pound of cheese please

Gaddy Ming
In sixteen flavours
Mouldy mounds
Wedding cake favours
Festering rabbits with skint knees
And a half pound of cheese please

A broken leg
Poke in the eye
Acne squeezing
In a meat pie
Artificial colouring for Xmas trees
And a half pound of cheese please

I wear a duffle coat
With elasticised garter
The shop is full of shoppers
Everyone a martyr

Here is my shopping list
Bag full of money
Come to get the shopping
Give it to my mummy

Daddy wears a funny hat
I hate my mummy
She can have the shopping list
I'll have the money
And a half pound of cheese please

The Incredible Invisible Woman

Has anyone seen Mrs Pollythene
The incredible invisible woman
Although she's never seen
She is very clean
Mrs Pollythene
The incredible invisible woman

She's got invisible eyes invisible nose
Invisible feet with invisible toes
Invisible hair with invisible bows
Where she lives nobody knows

She goes to the cinema and gets in free!
She goes to the football and gets in free!
She goes to the theatre and gets in free!
To be invisible I wish it were me!

She's married to a plastic bag
Who calls himself Bin Liner
Her friends are all double glazed
Nothing could be finer

Has anyone seen Mrs Pollythene

The incredible invisible woman

Although she's never seen

She is very clean

Mrs Pollythene

The incredible invisible woman

To her children she's transparent …

I Love To Go A Yodeling - 1977/2010 Hillbilly Mix

One, Two, Three

(Earl grey?) No that's gay
(Toast and jam?) Yes I can

Four, Five, Six
(Pick up sticks)

Seven, Eight, Nine
It's yodelling time...

I love to go a yodelling
It's a yodeller's life for me
I love to go a yodelling
And I love to drink my tea

I yodel in the wardrobe
I yodel in my pants
I yodel to my spider
And I yodel to my ants

(Chorus)

I yodel when I tap dance
With an earwig on each foot
I yodel in the brass band
And I yodel on the flute

I yodel in the bathroom
I yodel with my otter
I yodel when I'm in the shower
And I yodel underwater

(Chorus)

I yodel when I'm happy
I yodel when I'm sad
I yodel underneath the bed
And yodel with my dad

I yodel from the hilltops
I yodel with my mum
I yodel with your sister
She yodel's on my thumb

(Chorus)

I Wrestled a Worm

I saw a wrestler wrestling with a wrestler in the park
I'd rather wrestle wrestlers than wrestle in the dark

I saw an oarsman rowing with some oarsmen in a row
They were rowing with their oars why they were rowing I don't know

I saw a policeman policing with a policeman by his side
They were policing in a police car and I didn't want a ride
I saw a lumberjack lumber-jacking with a lumberjack called Jack
He was lumbering with some lumber with a lumberjack jacket on his back

I read the daily tabloids on the table with my tea
The *Telegraph* is terrifying it doesn't have page three

I saw a man from the Inland Revenue he didn't really like me
He said 'give me some money' I said 'not bloody likely'

He said 'you getting paid for that poem?'
I said 'what poem?'

Family Ties

Bet your bottom dollar
That your dime is upside down
Bet your sideways nickel
That your cent is half a crown

See your sister dancing
With a Maltese man in black
Gambling with his laundry
And your best friend's heart attack

Mother said don't speak to yourself
Isn't very easy when you're left on the shelf
Father said don't speak to the boys
They break your legs and steal your toys

If this is what they call family ties
I'd rather see through a dead man's eyes
If this what they call family games
I'd rather play with zombie's brains

I'm the king of the Bible class
I see the teacher and slap her ass
Jesus is cool he knows my dad
They eat fish suppers and I am glad

Silly Old Goat

Run like an antelope
Hop like a frog
Swim like an elephant
Fly like a dog

Silly old man silly old man
Lost his life in a watering can

Sick old donkey sick old goat
Have some fun and slit your throat

Run like a blackbird
Hop like a mouse
Swim like a monkey
Fly like a house

Silly old man silly old man
Lost his life in a watering can

Sick old donkey sick old goat
Have some fun and slit your throat

Mr Elastic Brain

Burn your boots

Burn your breeches

Cover your head

In luminous leeches

Big Tomato Plant

I wish
I was
A big tomato plant

Paste your yeti to the floor
Spread mayonnaise on the door

I wish
I was
A Mexican hot dog

Is that grated cheese entwined with your hairy chest?
Or a blancmange under your wig?

I wish
I was
A lemon soufflé

Black forest gateaux on the face
Greek salad in the ear

Is that a salmon sandwich behind your contact lens?

I wish
I was
A chicken casserole

Hay Babe
Is that a piece of salami strapped to your chin?

Well huh

I wish
I was
A big tomato plant

I wish
I was
Baked beans on toast

Baked beans on toast

Baked beans on toast

Tartan Underpants

They are groovy they can dance
They can put you in a trance
That's my tartan underpants
Tartan underpants ooh
Tartan underpants ooh

You can use them as a tent use then as a hanky
One thing is sure there's never hanky panky
In my tartan underpants
Tartan underpants ooh
Tartan underpants ooh

I don't drink whisky don't eat haggis
Go to bed with a girl from Paris
In my tartan underpants
Tartan underpants ooh
Tartan underpants ooh

My pants are funky they know what to do
Goodbye boxer shorts it's the Y-Front crew
That's my tartan underpants
Tartan underpants ooh
Tartan underpants ooh

I'm a boring old folk singer
Philip is my name
My mother is a miner
My sister's on the game

Mr Elastic Brain

I've a face like a scrotum
Wear an Arran jersey
Nobody likes me
I've got bad breath
Claymore !!!

My old sheep ran away
My dog is very angry
He hasn't slept all week
And likes a drink of shandy
Ben Nevis !!!

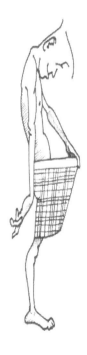

Salvador Dali's Hat

Robin Hood and his Merry Men
Robbed from the rich at half past ten
Gave to the poor at quarter past eight
They all said 'how's it going mate'?

Nicky nacky noo
What are you going to do?
I can do better than that
It's Salvador Dali's Hat

David and Goliath had a fight one day
Could have been April could have been May
One had a sword one had a sling
One was dead and the other was king

Nicky nacky noo
What are you going to do?
I can do better than that
It's Salvador Dali's Hat

King Arthur was a merry old sole
A merry old sole was he
Lancelot and Merlin at his table
Guinevere on his knee

Nicky nacky noo
What are you going to do?
I can do better than that
It's Salvador Dali's Hat

Romeo and Juliet up a tree
Kissing and snogaling I N Gee
Romeo got hot and took off his clothes
Along came a blackbird and pecked off his ...
Nose !

Nicky nacky noo
What are you going to do?
I can do better than that
It's Salvador Dali's Hat

Honky Tonk Banjo

They call me the Honky Tonk Banjo ... *yee ha!*

They call me the Honky Tonk Kid ... *yee hoo!*

With the woman and the song and the whisky and the gambling

They call me the Honky Tonk Kid ... *The Kid*

I was born in a freight train honey ... *whoo whoo!*

I was raised by a preacher man ... *hallelujah!*

I was schooled by some wild coyote

I take my beans from the can ... *from the can*

I made love to a cactus ... *oowh!!*

Dressed up like a buffalo ... *buffalo*

I used to ride shotgun on the stage-coach

To the injuns I'd say hello ... *hello!*

I brand myself like the cattle ... *aggh!*

They threw me out of the saloon ... *get out!*

Use a rock for a pillow

Bedside lamp is the moon ... *ahhoooo!*

I gargle bullets in the morning ... *p'ting!*

Smear horse manure on my chest ... *on his chest*

Rattlesnake lives in my long johns

Family of raccoon's up my vest ... *tickle tickle!*

They call me the Honky Tonk Banjo ... *yee ha!*

They call me the Honky Tonk Kid ... *yee hoo!*

With the woman and the song and the whisky and the gambling

I play my banjo with a tray ... *with a tray!*

Gran... Gran In A Frying Pan

Gran... Gran in a frying pan
Making macaroni, making macaroni
Gran... Gran in a frying pan
Making macaroni for the girls to eat

Och aye the noo!
My Granny caught a coo
She salted it and peppered it
And put it in a stew

Och michty me!
My Granny caught a flea
She salted it and peppered it
And had it for her tea

Oh diddely dum!
Her heed stuck up the lum
We'll salt her and we'll pepper her
And kick her up the bum

Gran... Gran in a frying pan

Making macaroni, making macaroni

Gran... Gran in a frying pan

Making macaroni for the girls to eat

Mr Wolfman

Excuse me
Are you Mr Potter today?
No
You wear that balaclava
Round the wrong way

Your Mr Wolfman
Awoo – awoo – awoo
Your Mr Wolfman
Awoo – awoo – awoo

Your life is like a shiny boot
Sore foot sore foot
Your trousers pressed your shirts are clean
So mean so mean
You drive a car your wear a tie
Not I not I
Your clean-cut image has to die
Not I not I
Eat your turnip eat your peas
No please no please
Wash your face and cut your hair
Not fair not fair
Your life is like a shiny boot
Sore foot sore foot

There once was a man called Potter
Who wanted a drink of water
He went down to the sea
And had a cup of tea
Instead of a drink of water

And he said

A funny thing happened to me
As I drank that cup of tea
Hair grew out every hole in me
Never again shall I watch TV
With hair growing out every hole in me

I'm Mr Wolfman
Awoo – awoo – awoo
I'm Mr Wolfman
Awoo – awoo – awoo

Sore foot

Free Sex Is A Go-Go VS Mr Glee And His Magic Flea

Inspiration flows thicker
In the veins of a bananahead
Said Millie Molly Mandy
To her mother who was dead

The devil is a woman and I met her last night
She said 'big boy let me give you a fright'
Well I'm not very big so she left me alone
Shortly after that I went on home

Walk on the sand
Hold hands with a monkey
Right eye boogie
Left eye funky

I've got a walking stick but I can walk
I've got a mouth but I can talk
I've got eyes but I can't see
The beauty in the girl and the beauty in me

I'm a virgin and I'm proud of it
I'm a virgin there's no doubt of it
Free sex free sex is a go-go
Free sex free sex is a new suit

Lived in a house lived in a tree
Do magic spells do some on me
Lived in a tent lived in the sea
Ha-ha-ha he-he-he it's Mr Glee and his magic flea

I knew a lady and she was very wobbly
She wobbled like a jelly as she fell down
Wobbled on the floor could not take any more
She broke my fingers and I was glad

I've a burning desire to set your house on fire
A burning desire to set your house on fire
When you're in the bushes trying to take a leak
It makes you nothing but a paranoid freak

Wheeze and sneeze and cough and splutter
Eat cold prawns with melted butter
Jump and leap and hop and stutter
Bananaman jive into the gutter

Lock yourself into a room
Hit your partner with a broom
Make a noise like a donkey
Time to go going wonky

The Spider And The Fly

Step into my parlour

Said the Spider to the Fly

How do you want me

Came the seductive reply

I'll lick you for my dinner

Lick you for my tea

And when it is suppertime

You can make love to me

New York – New York

New York - New York

So good

They named it

Arbroath – Arbroath

Arbroath – Arbroath

So good

They named

A fish after it

Monkeys Versus Donkeys

Monkeys versus Donkeys
Monkeys versus Donkeys
Monkeys versus Donkeys
Now

Take my Monkey
Race your Donkey
Monkey's going to win
Right now

Mickey the Monkey
He is very Funky
He's going to win
Right now

Look at your Donkey
He is very wonky
His mother is
A cow

Mickey is my Monkey
He can run so fast
Look at Mickey running
He has run right past

Look at your Donkey
Oh what a blast
Falls on his ass
And comes in last

Monkeys versus Donkeys
Monkeys versus Donkeys
Monkeys versus Donkeys

Now

Take my Monkey
Race your Donkey
Monkey's going to win
Right now

Red Hot Birthday Box

Let me play in your Red Hot Birthday Box

Re-ignite the flame

Your combustible elements of tenderness and rage

Dictate it will never be the same

Our ever present past

Darling help yourself

Help yourself Darling

I plunder your Red Hot Birthday Box

Play my favourite game

Quiet now Darling

Darling quiet now

Your mind is playing tricks on you

It's ok

Tomorrow you will live in colour

Amanda

White notes are enlightening

Black makes life exciting

Your music may sound serene

It's the spaces you leave between

That shows us your hidden light

Wonderfully dazzling on poetry night

People ask

What do you call that strange three-sided instrument?

And you say

Stanley!

After your late father

Who only ever wore a watch for decoration

Dublin City

When I was walking in Dublin City

I met a man called Walter Mitty

He was smart

And he was witty

But his underpants

Were slightly …………

……………… Pretty

The City Of Discovery

I discovered Camperdoon Park

Sunshine and circles

Pink-studded bitch belts

Twin buggies and matching roots

Fagging fag hags

Fagging fagging fags

In my fagging fase

Fagging fagging fag hags

Fag fags in your own fagging fase

Fag me

Fag you

Fag those

Fag knows

Fag on

Fag off

Fagging fagging fag hags

I discovered Camperdoon Park

Sunshine and circles

Pink-studded bitch belts

Twin buggies and matching roots

The City of Discovery

What a pleasant surprise

Yesterday

Yesterday

I was told

That when you are our age

And lucky enough

To have an erection

You should always use it

This morning

I used mine

To draw a straight line

It was a very long line

But

Not very

Straight

Scarlet Harlot

Scarlet Harlot pudding and pie

Kissed the boys and made them die

When all the funds had gone away

Scarlet Harlot made them pay

And pay

And pay

Everyone has an emotional need

She fills her vacuum with emotional greed

Every day is a Doris Day day

Co-dependant happiness the Rock Hudson way

Shoot the crow and kill the cock

The cow ran away with my grandfather's clock

Like Barbarella and Rockefeller

Keeps herself locked up in the cellar

She'll do you nightly like Holly Golightly

The golden butterfly with the scorpion sting

Douglas John McLean Cairns

Butterfly butterfly where have you been?
I've been to London to visit the Queen
Butterfly butterfly what did you do there?
I saw a hole in the ozone layer

Scarlet Harlot pudding and pie
Kissed this boy
and made
him
cry

Margot

Margot you thought I forgot
To put the T into Margo
Oh no I did not forgo
The O in Margot

Margot J Cairns

People ask you what the J stands for
And you say J
Jay A Y
And they say why

And you say
It's lest you forgot
Your father was an idiot
Margot J Cairns

Adam and Eve

Adam and Eve, Cane and Abel
Sat down one day at the kitchen table
They had loafs and they had fishes
Along came an angel and did the dishes

Let's Rock!

Sputnik Sweetheart Strawberry Tart

Sputnik sweetheart strawberry tart
Who's the man who's got your heart?
Is he a bad man?
Is he a sad man?
Is he a man without any teeth?

I met a pretty Russian Girl from St Petersburg
Stunned by her honesty
She came to my room
Drank green tea
Read my poetry
Looked stunned
Shook hands

And left

Sputnik sweetheart strawberry tart
Who's the man who's got your heart?
Is he a bad man?
Is he a sad man?
Is he a man without any teeth?

I met a pretty Russian Girl from St Petersburg
She asked me why I had never made a move
I suggested the Foxtrot
Realising it may be acceptable to occupy some of her
personal space
I mumbled
I'm scared
She held my hand
It was warm and soft

So was I

Sputnik sweetheart strawberry tart
Who's the man who's got your heart?
Is he a bad man?
Is he a sad man?
Is he a man without any teeth?

I met a pretty Russian Girl from St Petersburg
I kissed her in Rembrandt's house
She suggested next time I try the lips
A female member of security
Leapt from the shadows
Kissing is not acceptable in a house of fine art
Sorry I thought this was the kissing museum
Wrong!!

She had cobwebs in her underpants!

John O Groats

Folks from John O Groats
When in boats
Wear floats
Around their throats
But don't have notes
In their coats
Giving safety instructions

But

Folks from John O Groats
When in moats
Don't have floats
Around their throats
But have notes
In their coats
Giving directions home
The answer is normally

North

A Giraffe's Tale

Tall Paul Giraffe sat in a bath
Blowing bubbles out of his bum
Along came his mum who stuck in a thumb
Said stop that you'll go blind

Pardon me for being so rude
It was not me it was my food
It popped out to say hello
On the south wind down below

It's OK it smells of roses
That's why giraffes have big long noses
Twenty feet from their tail
Lucky it's not a dung-eating snail

They create an horrendous smell
Kept inside their tiny shell
Exploding by the light of the moon
Unless eaten by a poor baboon

Swinging from tree to tree
Serenading a Mexican flea
Exploding snails inside their tums
That's why baboons they have big red bums

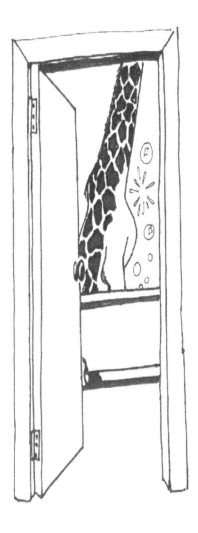

Fish

Fish fish fish fish

Fishy fishy fish foo

Fish fish fish fish

Fishy fishy flop floo

Fish fish fish fish

Fishy fishy fish fish

Fish fish fish fish

Fishy fishy flip flop

Fish fish fish fish

Fishy fishy fish fin

Fish fish fish fish

Fishy fishy flip floop

Mmmm...

I think something fishy's going on

Splish splash splish splash

Splashy splashy splish splash

Splish splash splish splash

Splishy splashy poo

Haddock in a Mist
Aftershave ... for MEN

Lazy Lion

Lazy lion
Lying all around
Laying on the grass
Laying on the ground
Laying on the sofa
Laying on the bed
Laying on top of the elephant's head

Oh said the Zebra that's not fair
Now that elephant's got lots of hair
Look at me I'm bald and stripy
No problem said the lion
Who got all bitey

Oh said the Zebra
Let go of my leg
No problem said the Lion
You'll soon be dead
I'll be a lazy old lion
Laying on the sofa
Laying on the bed
Laying on top of the elephant's head

I Am Amsterdam

Five Dollar Pete
With his size ten feet

Stanley Knife
With his two foot wife

Mike Stand
With his elastic band

Tam Boreen
With his groovy scene

Jimmy Shoo
With his Asian flu

Amsterdam Annie
With her …

Entrepreneurial Endeavours & Monthly Government
Health Checks

I've Got A Rocking Chair

I've got a rocking chair

It Rocks

I've got a sock

It Socks

Me on the jaw

Like an old American movie

Often seen on TV

With Adam West and his batman vest

And Robin

Who just sort of hangs around

A bit like

A scrotum

You Woke Me Up

You woke me up and took my dream away

It only comes out on a sunny day

I will have to lay still

Wait till next summer

Living in Rainy Scotland

Can sometimes be

A bummer …

Douglas John McLean Cairns

Third Bit

Tip Top - Sid Ozalid

Gig Review

Douglas John McLean Cairns

The Artist Formally Known as Sid Ozalid

Poetry Café - Covent Garden – London Town
September 2010

When in London town I thought it a good idea to go perform at the Poetry Café in Covent Garden. They have an open mic night on Tuesdays called Poetry Unplugged. Not wishing to appear as an out of towner, I walked to the Poetry Café on the Monday evening to ensure I knew its location.

A marvellous eight-minute walk from my accommodation, overlooking the London Eye on the embankment. It was a five-minute return journey, there was a heavy down pour of rain and I had no jacket with me. I also stepped in a very deep puddle of water at traffic lights when trying to avoid a waterfall of many colours that was directed my way from a nice red London bus.

Tuesday night, gig night. Interested poets have to 'sign on' between 18.00 and 19.00. In preparation I wrote out the address of the Poetry Café on a yellow sticky and printed out a few poems, that I thought may fit in well amongst the learned folks of London town. Wishing to impress with my personal hygiene, I hopped in the shower and ran through my poems for the evening.

I left the embankment at 17.55 and struck out for the Poetry Café; it would be my first time on stage in years. Still no jacket but feeling rather focused I took a wrong turning and started to go round and round in circles. The journey had become more and more confusing as I wandered along brightly-lit streets filled with noise and tourists. I was getting more and more confused. I longed to be at home in my croft with my invisible friends:

Jimmy the Sheep, Robert the Cat and Micky the Monkey, who is not invisible but a very good friend.

This was when I remembered that if you are going to write out the address in advance, it is a good idea to take it with you. Silly foolish boy!

If you want directions, ask a policeman. I asked two separate policemen. Both had no idea what I was talking about and said that this was their first night working in the area of Covent Garden. It must be a rough area if policemen only last one night and have to be changed out or laid to rest, like sleeping policemen.

I did see Mike Jones from the Clash walking past and was rather scooped; he was with some young dude with cool hair, otherwise he may have rushed over and asked for my autograph and given me directions. But I did not want to embarrass him in front of his young friend, and after all he had his chance of an autograph in 1977 and again in 1982 so why make it third time lucky.

I did find the venue, by asking in another café. Turned out I was 30 seconds from it, but was getting more and more confused and had left my medication and directions at home. Better still when I arrived at 19.15 and saw the place full of poets reading over their work, it dawned on me that I had also left my poems behind.

The kind organising man let me sign on late, but I was told that I was very lucky and this would not always be aloud. I was to be on in the second half.

Coffee and cake in hand I sat at the back of the room as it filled up with interesting people. It got darker and darker and hotter and hotter. Turns out that 25 poets would perform with 5 minutes per poet. I was in need of an oxygen tent, pacemaker and a rub down with my favourite silk scarf. Mmm…. Silk!

Each poet got up in turn reading their stunning work, plugging their next gig or selling their latest book. I started to think that staying at home and watching Scotland play football very very badly could have been much better for my health and heart rate. I had no book, no next gig and could not remember any words to any of my own work.

Still two and a half hours in a hot dark room is nothing new to me. Turns out the second half was just as good as the first half, but I did not know when I would be on. These poets were great… and I was in line for a heart attack.

As a Poetry Café virgin I thought they would sling me on stage in between some recognised poets, just in case I was a mumbling fool. Turns out through a strange game of giving each poet a nick name related to some sort of monster character and letting the audient pick … I was on last. After Dracula, Woolfman and Hunchback.

The audience thought I was very funny, not because I was, but because I had told them that I had got lost, left the directions behind as well as my poetry and had asked two policemen for directions. Lucky for me I did not share the fact that it took me over and hour to get there and I had checked it out very successfully the night before. They may well have asked me to sit back down till they phoned a cab to take me home.

After spending an evening hearing poetry delivered by some of London's best. I think my renditions of *'Red Eared Seagull'*, *'I Wrestled a Worm'* and *'Stepping Out'* took them a bit by surprise. Not may people had delivered their poems with accompanying body, arm and hand movements. But not all the poets had given dance classes to the Queen.

I have the pleasure to report that people really enjoyed my performance and lots of clapping was done to accompany the laughing and smiling faces. People shook my hand and offered to sort me out 'upstairs'. This turned out to be an offer of a beverage of my own choice at the upstairs café. I declined, but in a nice way. Did not want to get to close to those London Poetry types.

Feeling somewhat pleased with myself, I struck out with new confidence, and took another wrong turning. This time cutting it down to a one-hour wander round some very interesting dark streets of London. Some nice young men who called themselves a 'posse' stopped me in the street and asked where I had got my shirt from as they would also like a garment of such fine stature. I explained that I got it in Holland for my birthday and that it may not be available in London town. The young men suggested that they remove it from my person for their own use. My goodness! Word of my performance had spread faster than the fire of London and people were not only content with shaking my hand but now wanted a bit of the Ozalid wardrobe.

It only took me a few seconds to explain to the young gents, that as nice as it was of them to follow me into a dark underpass I would need to keep my shirt as I had no vest or indeed jacket to keep me warm. We exchanged some strange dialogue, theirs being a variety I would imagine could be found in the streets of London town and my more poetic but surprisingly aggressive overtones being somewhat more of the Scottish variety. The young men kindly left once they understood that as large as I am, the four of them would never fit into my shirt.

Back in my room the adrenalin was still flowing so I decided to entertain the mini bar. Once all the food and drink was finished I felt it only proper to visit the Japanese gent in the next room and tell him I was the hotel mini-bar inspector who had been sent to remove the content of his mini-bar for the evening and would return next morning with some free tickets and a yellow sticky giving directions to the Poetry Café.

On my return home to Holland I found out that I had left my bike keys some place in the UK and could not cycle home from the station, but the important thing was that I still had the shirt on my back and a bag full of donkeys for the kids.

Viva Sid!!
Viva London Town!!
And more importantly …
Viva Teflon non-stick underpants!!

Love, Peace and light …

The Artist Formally known as Sid Ozalid xx

The End

Douglas John McLean Cairns

Fourth Bit

Some other Stuff

Douglas John McLean Cairns

List of people who have performed with Sid on stage

Jeremy Thoms Sam	Phil Craig Guitar
Frieda Munro Wig	George Norval Stuff
Colin Maclean Drum	Gerry 'Bongo' Dawson Trumpet and vibes
Darryl Thomson Keys	Alex Lovie More stuff and noise
Jennifer Ann Coconut Wig	David McLeod Seeing is believing
Andi Holbrook Bass	Fiona McKinnon Sid's Mum
Colin Jenkins Freak	Sheena Dixon Puppets
Eoghan Howard Bass	Roy Gott Legs
John Todd Bass	Shona Reppe More puppets

List of people who are no longer with Sid

I have been very lucky to have had so many people help me with my performances over the years, the list is very long and I cannot remember everyone. I would like to take the time to remember and thank those who have passed away and who made a special effort to support me along my journey as Sid.

Sheena Dixon
Puppeteer

Paddy Burns
Comedian and friend

Marline Ross
Friend

Kate Marx
Friend

Bruce Kennedy
DJ

Henry Morrice
Friend

John Cairns
Father

Acknowledgements

Some people have had to put up with me writing this book. I thank them from the bottom of my socks.

Thank you Anna for letting me use the dining room table for more than just dining.

Thank you John Angus McLeod of the clan McLeod for helping me chose the poetry content and helping with the photos.

Thank you to Donald Smart for the groovy cartoons you can find him at smartcaricatures.co.uk.

Thank you to Claire Haugh for all the professional editing advice, you have a wonderful red pen.

Thanks also to my Mum and Dad, just for being you and being cool. I love you both very much.

The Artist Formally Known As Sid Ozalid

If you are interested in finding out more about Sid Ozalid or hearing him perform some of the poems in this book, you can find him on Facebook.com and YouTube.com or down your local supermarket sticking fake moustaches onto pineapples.

SidOzalid.com

Lightning Source UK Ltd.
Milton Keynes UK
UKOW040038290413

209918UK00001B/2/P